Painting with
the Clouds

Painting with the Clouds

Life Before, During, and After Alzheimer's Disease

Charles R. McCain Ph.D.
&
Celeste Barefield RN, BSN

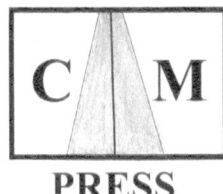

PRESS

P.O. Box 1096
Denison, TX

Cover photograph by
David Jones
Metairie, LA.

ISBN: 1517596599
ISBN 13: 9781517596590
Library of Congress Control Number: 2015916237
CreateSpace Independent Publishing Platform
North Charleston, South Carolina

FOR HELEN

Introduction

THIS IS AN account of a portion of our lives with Alzheimer's, the artist, the nurse, and the professor, all with the complications from Alzheimer's Disease. Helen was my mother; she's the artist. Charles is her husband, and he's the professor.

Mom had the misfortune to develop Alzheimer's; we all suffered from it. We have shared our journey through the good and the bad of it all. We even share the very end to try to give hope to those of you asking yourself what will this disease do to us? What will the end be like? Is there life after Alzheimer's?

We've included some short notes she wrote and emails between us trying to make the best quality of life for her. We will share our joys and our pains now. We hope, dear reader, that our authentic feelings and the results of all our efforts will help you, especially if you have to walk down this rocky road.

Celeste Barefield, RN, BSN

Charles R. McCain, Ph.D.

Contents

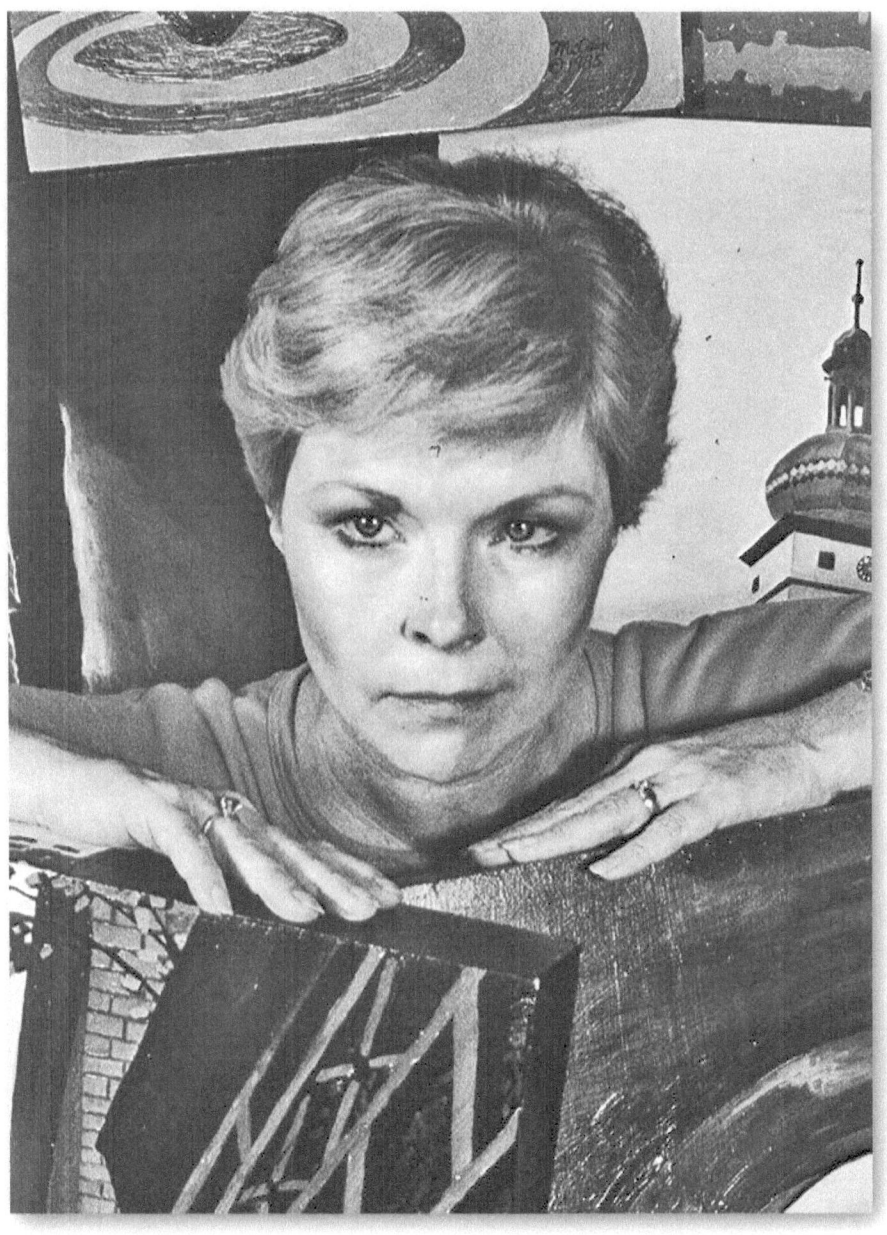

Helen Louise (Goff) McCain
1938 - 2014

PART 1

All the King's Horses

As I SIT at my kitchen table viewing the beautiful sunset, I realize how tired I am. I have been doing this for two days, and I know that this is not doing me any good. I must rejoin the world. I also realize that it will be such a difficult task without her, my love and my life.

Only God could have saved her from the terrible disease of dementia. She struggled as best as she could those final days of almost a living death. I'm not sure it is in me to describe what I witnessed. It is well beyond me even to recollect how much a human being can so quickly slip from normality to an unrecognizable person who was once a wonderful, kind, and loving wife who doted on me as if I were a king. But I will try for the sake of those yet to come.

Oh me, oh my! Producing this account of her "journey" will be a huge challenge.

First, there is no cure for dementia (as far as I know), at least by 2015. All her doctor could do is to make the journey as comfortable as possible. By the time she was diagnosed with dementia, some excellent medications had come on the market, and these "meds" had to be prescribed by medical doctors. So I can honestly say that everything possible was done to try and stabilize her condition until the disease finally overcame even the best meds that the pharmaceutical industry and medical science had to offer. Knowing this day-by-day that she had a terminal disease did not raise my spirits by being her caregiver. It's sort of like watching a beautiful candle eventually burn until no wax remains. And then the flame on the wick gently flickers, then goes out.

Her kind demeanor is what I will miss the most. Most of the time she was marvelously positive, almost childlike but in an adult way. If I had asked her, she would be the first to admit she had not lived a sterling life before she married me. I paid little attention to that statement because neither had I; I considered her to have behaved as a human being like most of us do day by day.

This story is told in retrospect although I have some emails from family and friends to help relate the psychological impact on some family members' day to day life.

This story actually begins about 1991. That's where I begin.

PART 2

Into The Breach

HELEN WAS BUSY planning the evening meal when I left for work that March morning in 1991. The day before had been holy hell for her -- she had another bout with migraine headaches. It was getting apparent that so far doctors were puzzled about what to do to stop them. About all they did was prescribe painkillers which could be addictive. She hated that because she couldn't drive her new car in that condition, so she tolerated the headaches so she could drive and get out of the house. Frankly, I don't know how she did it.

Many days I returned home from work to find a note telling me she had another "headache" and put my "supper" in the fridge or the oven. Her condition had been worsening for a few weeks, and only a couple of months before did she seek out a doctor for help.

Dr. Jergensen examined her and said the headaches should go away in a relatively short time, perhaps a couple of weeks or so. She had told him she had been in an automobile accident when she was a young girl and had been "knocked out" for a few minutes. During the years since, she had experienced a headache now and then but attributed them to daily living. Only in the last six months had the pain elevated to the severe level. It was then when she sought out a doctor.

When she had one of those headaches, she requested total silence and a dark room. She would feel a migraine coming on before the severe pain came, so sometimes one of her pills would lessen the pain. By 1993, however, some of the strongest medications did little good. Her best bet was to go to bed and try to sleep away the headache. *Sometimes* that worked.

By that time, we seldom went out except to a restaurant when she felt okay. I think we went "out" at times even though she didn't feel well. She was not selfish, and sometimes she "bit the bullet" and didn't tell me she had a headache. But she wanted to do things out of the house. Only a few years before we had made summer trips to the Western United States to see interesting places like Taos, New Mexico and the Grand Canyon. In 1988 we drove through several Southeastern states all the way to South Carolina and back through Alabama where we stopped for a couple of days while I visited the county court house and the local public library to find records on my family in the 1800s. We also drove to Atlanta to meet with my long lost cousins. Yes, I had become interested in family history in a big way. I have stayed with it until the present day.

I think we had a good life even with her headache problem. My salary allowed us to attend several concerts, ballets, and musical productions. At the time, we lived in a suburb of Dallas, Texas.

I retired from college teaching in 1994, and we moved to the countryside near Denison, Texas where her widowed mother lived. Helen's mother had about 25 acres of land, so she told Helen she could have about nine acres next door. It was Helen's legacy, and we put our roots down there and began our retired life.

That part of Grayson County is, in my opinion, the prettiest part of the state with many Post Oak trees. Even in the years of drought, these rugged trees survived the tremendous temperatures and lack of rain during the hot Texas summers. There is a Post Oak tree in our back lot. It must be 100 years old and about 100 feet tall.

So starting in 1995 she and I went through her siege of terrible migraine headaches. She must have gone through several local doctors who seemed to be clueless about what to do except throw pills at the problem. She even was treated by two so-called local neurologists who seemed to be just as puzzled. We were both beginning to believe that most doctors are so ego-driven that they wouldn't admit they didn't know how to treat severe migraine headaches.

That's when I began investigating the problem on the Internet on sites of respectable medical institutions. That opened an entirely new world of possibilities. I quickly was able to confirm that most of the migraine medications were not effective, and I began to think of the thousands of dollars we had spent on ineffective prescriptions. During this period, the medical insurance company had complained bitterly at the cost of the medications as well as the frequency to refill them. The insurance people claimed by their contract with my original organization that they were not obligated to approve the number and frequency of refilling the medications. That's when I began to look for another doctor. The hassle by the insurance people finally took its toll. I was exhausted trying to work with the fiscal conservatives who only had the bottom line of their company in mind. They didn't give a damn about the patient.

But one good procedure did come out of all those doctor visits – she was directed to have an MRI on her brain that produced evidence of tiny "dots" called TIAs (please don't ask me what TIA means). In non-medical terms, it seemed to mean that she had experienced tiny heart problems (strokes). The doctor said she had them without knowing it. It is possible that the TIAs could have influenced the coming on of dementia?

But knowing about the TIAs seemingly did nothing to help with dealing with the problem. She had been seeing this neurologist for almost four years. My reaction was that he didn't know what to do and was just collecting fees. In the warm late Summer of 2009, I contacted a Dallas doctor. It seems the doctors around here were not able to help Helen.

Fortunately for us, Helen's daughter, Celeste, is a registered nurse, and she too began making inquiries about the problem. She came up with a Dr. Lewis in Dallas who specialized in her problem. At Helen's first appointment in August, 2009, Dr. Lewis cancelled most of her then current medications and wrote new ones. One was Aricept which immediately helped because I could see Helen stabilizing into a semblance of her old self. It seems Dr. Lewis was really a specialist in dementia! At the next appointment, he prescribed Namenda which worked well with Aricept. Without a doubt, the dementia had been stabilized, but it was to be only a band-aid. The meds did work, and that meant a lot. The migraines had mostly gone away. Helen could take over-the-counter meds to help her headaches. They had dwindled to only an occasional problem which she could handle. That left dementia that Dr. Lewis had diagnosed. At that point, Alzheimer's disease had not been mentioned by the doctor.

PART 3

Slippery Slope

BEING A CAREGIVER for a dementia patient includes many duties other than ensuring his/her patient has what is needed day to day. Here is a general example:

Imagine two people living together sharing the household chores as well as those outside like keeping the lawn mowed, home repairs inside and out, *etc*. Now imagine that one of the persons is no longer able to complete most of those duties. Now realize that someone, a member of the household or not, has to assume the chores. Those added duties fall upon the caregiver to make sure these duties are completed. This can be a heavy burden. Most middle class households cannot afford to hire someone to pick up these chores, so the work falls on the caregiver one way or the other.

Sunday, March 21, 2010 -- Helen has had the dementia symptoms for over four years, but the progress of the disease has been very slow. Each person must have one's antenna up to detect the symptoms or warning signs. In my case, I did not. Any changes I detected I attributed to age or the effects of her terrible migraine headaches several months before. It was not until 2009 did I even become aware of changes in her behavior, and that was due to Celeste who told me one day that Helen had dementia. It didn't register clearly with me immediately. As a matter of fact, it was at least a month before the weight of the pronouncement actually hit me . . . hard!

I can now look back and see what was happening right in front of me; I **did not** notice then. Unfortunately I can't go back and change a thing!

Today is a red-letter day for me. I noted some real changes in her behavior. On one hand she has shown the proclivity to forget events that happened only a few days ago; on the other hand she can clearly remember many events that happened prior to 1982. At one time she lived in New Orleans and another in Boston. She can remember names as well as events. But today I was saddened to find out that that most of our married life is a blank slate. She doesn't remember our wedding or any of the events up to the present. I learned this in conversation with her. Further, she has to ask my full name once in a while, sometimes daily.

She looked at me puzzled when I told her we have been married all these years. She said, "No, I don't think so." Fortunately, I have many photos of the wedding on my computer, so I printed several for her. Her daughter and friends were there with a younger version of both of us with all our friends. She carefully looked over the photos, and said, "I guess we are married then! I thought you were just a good friend of the family. But now I understand."

Next week, she will not remember all this, and I may have to repeat what I did today. Is this distressing to me? Damn right it is! It is so sad that the memories of all those good years are lost forever. So I try to make good memories for her each day by letting her have her way when possible. She enjoyed going to restaurants, so we went out when she wanted to go.

My goal in all this was to make her time with me as pleasant as I could even though I knew the eventual outcome.

Looking back, it all seems like a blur. But I know that I can remember most everything in reasonable detail. The earliest indications of Alzheimer's displayed by Helen were not noticed by me. Celeste, told me that she suspected Helen was developing dementia as early as 2007. Of course looking back I can see now what I didn't see then. One of the earliest signs she displayed a memory problem. One day in 2008 she came home and related that she had taken so long because she forgot her route home. She said that the people at the store were very understanding and helped her find her way back home by giving her good directions. I didn't take a great deal of notice to that, but I wondered what was going on.

For some time she had not resumed painting, and I wondered about that. She seemed to enjoy that so much. At the same time she ceased doing any sewing even though she had a very good sewing machine. She would sit and her easy chair and make napkins by hand from pieces of cloth, but that seemed to be the extent of her sewing. I wondered about that too.

Finally in 2008 she really began to show memory problems. For example, she was an expert cook, and I emphasize the word *expert*. I know that cooking was one of the more pleasant activities that she did. One evening she served me food that was either undercooked or overcooked. It was so unlike her cooking. Up to that point the food she prepared was excellent. I asked her what the problem was, and she said she had forgotten some of her recipes and how long to cook food. Unfortunately that evening the food was not edible, so I suggested we go out to eat. She did not argue with me. I don't remember where we went, but I never did throw that up to her because I knew she was very embarrassed. However from then on she made many mistakes in cooking. I helped as much as I could in the kitchen. My solution was to go out.

My recollection of that period of time is the last that she was able to prepare a really good meal which she had done for so many years. Even if I suggested that we go out, she always said, "My food is better." And it was or had been.

And, as I recall, that period was the beginning of subtle changes in her personality. She began to display traits of a person who was not happy is the best I can describe her at the time. Celeste has written a much better account of her psychological profile and how she behaved. I was actually awestruck at times because I did not know how to handle the situation. Had I been much more sensitive to her moods, I think I could've handled everything much better. I became rather passive in my dealings with her; I decided not to challenge or correct her when she made mistakes. By 2009, she was telling me I was not her husband and at times asked me to go home because she was a single lady. How all that went down is fairly well described and Celeste's account of the progression of this disease.

In retrospect, I honestly believe I did all that I could based on what I knew. I had no experience with dementia or Alzheimer's disease, so when I came across these symptoms, I blindly ignored them. It is my hope that as more information is available about dementia that people will be more sensitive and able to handle the situation better than I did.

My answer was to take her to specialists to assist with her problem. After all has been said and done, I am convinced that many of these specialists had no idea what they were doing when it came to Migraine headaches. Two local doctors led me on a wild goose chase while they "experimented" with various medications which did absolutely no good at all. Not to mention the angst, we spent literally thousands of dollars for zero help. I can only hope as the 21st century goes on that these specialists will become educated about Migraines and Alzheimer's disease and how to treat patients humanly or refer them to someone who could.

PART 4

My Cup Runneth Over

MY FAMILY PHYSICIAN told me that being the only caregiver for an Alzheimer's patient would catch up to me sooner or later. He advised me to find a nursing home locally. At first I felt like I would be a turncoat to do that, but deep down I knew it was a wise move.

Seeing my doctor was the culmination of several events, all of which were very stressful. After the episodes with the local sheriff, I knew I could not watch her 24/7. There were quite a few other occurrences that led up to my decision.

Some of these events happened only once, but others repeated. Once, when she claimed I was not her husband, I nearly lost it because she said she was a single lady. It all goes back to memory.

She wrote countless "notes" to me, leaving them at various places in the house. Some made no sense but other notes accused me of various crimes such as kidnapping and attempting murder via poison. Her paranoia at that time was rampant and very difficult to deal with. My only saving grace was being very calm and deliberate and speaking in a mild, non-threatening voice. At one point Celeste said she was worried Helen might do me harm, especially while I slept. I have a double lock on my front door which requires a key to open it from either side. That *only* ensured that she could not "escape"; the back door is set up the same. There are no side doors. Fortunately her meds helped her sleep through the night, so I didn't worry much about what she might do at night. But I always slept with one eye open.

After a visit with a doctor there were usually small changes in the meds which sometimes required a degree of negotiation on my part. Yes, she had Alzheimer's, but she was not stupid. And I always told her if this or that pill was new (she usually didn't remember going to a doctor which made my job more difficult). Being even-handed and patient, I usually was successful.

Being her caregiver was, without a doubt, the most difficult job I ever undertook. If she took a nap, so did I because I didn't know when I would have the next opportunity. Rest for a caregiver is essential. I always feared I might give Helen the wrong med at the wrong time due to exhaustion, so I placed a high priority on getting rest whenever the opportunity came.

There were a few rational moments. She would help me with the grocery list when the time came. But the hard part when it was time to go to the store. Sometimes she indicated no interest in going with me; I had to cajole her, using the epitome of diplomacy before leaving the house. There wasn't anyone for me to call and ask for help in this matter. All the family lived at least 100 miles away; it was up to me to get the job done.

I would wait until a favorite food or snack ran out; when she asked why we didn't have something, I'd tell her that if she would come with me to the store, she could pick out what she wanted. This usually worked. In the store, I had to be sure she stayed with me after she picked out her choices; then I could collect the items we needed for our meals. I cannot emphasize the importance of keeping an eye on her at that time. She could have easily been distracted and walked out the door without my noticing. That could have been disastrous.

After the events involving law enforcement, I finally realized that I could no longer handle the situation. Celeste and I discussed what we needed to do -- find a local nursing home. We did. Helen had been committed to a psychiatric facility in town to determine her needs. At that time, her medications were assessed and corrected. From there she was taken via ambulance to the nursing home quite a distance from my home. Later we moved her to one much nearer where she stayed until her death.

Altogether she was ill with the disease for 9-10 years, not knowing exactly when the disease took hold for sure. All Celeste and I knew is when the strange behavior began. Helen could have developed the disease for at least ten years.

PART 5

The Die Is Cast

THESE ARE MY final comments about caring for Helen. The question begs: "Would I do anything differently?" The answer is a definite YES. On one hand, if I had known how and what to do in the beginning, I probably would have behaved differently. On the other hand, I would not have been able to spend as much time with her if I had sent her to a nursing home early on.

I think nursing homes overall do a good job caring for dementia residents. At first, Helen did not want to stay at her new home. I visited at least twice a week (sometimes more often). For at least three months, she pleaded with me to take her back home. My answer was that I could not care for her as well as the nurses could where she was. That usually did not dampen her desire to return home.

During the first year I checked her out of the nursing home and brought her home where she immediately was able to remember the chair where she sat in the living room and the bed where she slept, although she never stayed the night. At other times I took her to her favorite restaurant (Chinese food); at other times Celeste drove in, and we all went to a restaurant.

Helen showed less interest in those activities during the 2nd and third year in the nursing home. She told me she liked the food in the nursing home, and begged off when I asked her if she wanted to go out to a restaurant. From then on she did not leave the facility.

Before selecting a place for her, I made sure that the unit for dementia patients was secured by a locked door with a key pad so nurses, other personnel, and visitors could enter and leave. My decision was correct because I had read where dementia patients walked out of a nursing home and either became lost or seriously injured on the outside. There were a number of horror stories on this subject in the media.

I was fortunate that I had carefully saved over the years and was able to secure Helen a place in a decent nursing home. And there are families who are financially strapped and have a very difficult time affording sending a loved one to a nursing home. But nearly every county in the country has an agency serving senior citizens. In my case, our local agency on the elderly was of great help in furnishing me with good information where to find assistance. I had to hire an elder care attorney (which was expensive), but he helped me secure financial help to ensure Helen was properly cared for in a nursing home.

This ends my story that lasted several years. Helen died a while back, and now I have no one to visit. I miss my times with her so much, even if she was ill. She is *the* love of my life, and I know we will be together again in the Hereafter.

PART 6

And the Band Played On

ALL THE EVENTS thus mentioned led up to 2009 when Helen's disease became more evident, albeit very slowly. As her husband and caregiver, I was oblivious to most of the "clues" of this terrible disease's beginnings. After seeing several so-called local specialists for about a year, I became rather negative to the idea that doctors could help her. I noted subtle changes in her behavior over that year, but I felt helpless until her daughter, Celeste, suggested early symptoms of dementia.

Over the period of 2009-2010, doctors prescribed many medications as though they were experimenting to see what worked. After her bout with severe headaches, I was beginning to have serious doubts about just what the medical people really knew.

In late 2009 she developed a skin condition that caused severe itching. I took her to a local dermatologist who diagnosed the condition and prescribed Cyproheptad and Hydrozyzine in addition to her other meds: Premarin, folic acid, Methotrexate, Namenda, and Effexor XR. I had to be on hand all day everyday to ensure she took these meds at the prescribed times.

About that time, Celeste, being a registered nurse, took her to an Alzheimer specialist in Dallas, Texas. That's when things began to change. From the first appointment, Dr. Lewis was highly suspicious Helen had the disease. He cancelled most of her current medications and added Aricept. That along with Namenda seemed to help her more than anything in the past.

Dr. Lewis, however, had a very poor bedside manner which seemed to upset Helen considerably and asked if a new doctor could be found. Fortunately Celeste knew of someone, Dr. Hurlinger, also in that area.

Painting with the Clouds

During her first visit with Dr. Hurlinger, Helen was given many tests. During the second appointment he told her he was confident she suffered from dementia. She was not very accepting of the diagnosis and complained for months afterward. It seems denial is common with dementia patients when first told the news.

Many emails continued from then on between Celeste and me. Throughout this treatise, parts of these communications will be shared with you, the reader, so you will begin to develop a concept of what it is like to have a loved one with this disease.

After the diagnoses by the last two doctors, I then knew what the eventual outcome would be. Up to that time Helen, on one hand, could be her same "old self"; on the other hand, she could also be a virago (shrew), showing signs of paranoia. As time went on, the former behavior lessened, and the latter began to dominate. As I got through this morass of behaviors, she would have called the local sheriff three times, accusing me of attempting to murder her by various means. All during this time, she claimed she was a single lady, and I was one of several men who came and went each day. At night, she suffered from "sun downing", a condition which compounded the dementia because the patient was tired after a long day.

Caring for a dementia patient is challenging at best. I had no training to equal this task. Fortunately for me, my daughter is a registered nurse. She guided me through many of my duties. Every day I thanked God for her suggestions. She came often to visit her Mom and me although it was a great inconvenience to her. I believe Celeste was the main reason I was able to get through being Helen's caregiver. But I would do it again in a New York minute.

PART 7

Give Me Anything But Reality

BEING THE CAREGIVER for Helen turned out to be very complicated. Her daily needs were great even aside from handing out medications. I became provider of the food (eat in or out), keeping clothes washed, errand boy, and a host of other little jobs. Much of the time during the day she behaved well; as the night drew near that usually changed. Once after 8 PM she wanted me to turn off the TV because she said the networks had hidden cameras in the TV screen to spy on us. The first time that happened, I did turn off the TV, but about five minutes later she became bored and retired to the bedroom for the night.

In early 2010, a problem with her meds came up, so I emailed Celeste: --- On **Sat, 3/20/10,** I wrote:

Dear Celeste:

When Helen got up today, she wanted me to change her meds because she was experiencing a lot of "singing" in her head. She said it was so distracting that sometimes she had a difficult time having a conversation. I believe her because only God knows what her brain is doing to her. Or that could mean her disease has taken a big step further. I don't know what's going on, and I won't know until she sees her doctor. Our dermatologist, Dr. Kantor, said she could discontinue taking Cyproheptad and Hydroxyzine because her skin condition had improved (he didn't see her lower back and buttocks). So she said she wanted me to continue the two which I had not given her this week. So this morning I added them to her pill caddy. I am confident those two meds will not

harm her since she has taken them for over a year. In a couple of days I'll ask her if she is still experiencing the "singing". You might say that she is "between" doctors right now, so I will have to consult with our family doctor if the issue comes up again. Love, Dad

Celeste's response was:

Lexapro, her depression medicine, will cause her head to "sing" if she misses taking it. She picks at her skin out of habit now I believe, but I don't think she has much itching now; or she may. She is probably complaining out of habit too; it's what she does.

These communications occurred almost daily because I wanted Celeste to know everything that went on related to her Mom's disease. After the "singing" episode, Helen didn't complain about taking her depression med. As a matter of fact, she became rather cooperative on that score *most of the time*!

I kept fairly close contact with parts of the family such as my two first cousins located in other states which are more than 1,000 miles away. June and Ellen were most interested in Helen's journey and asked if I would keep them in the loop. I did, and they were quick to respond.

On June 7, I wrote to Judy:

When I attended the Alzheimer's Meeting yesterday, I learned that (*legally*) Helen can no longer drive, according to the Texas Driving Code. I hated to tell her that, but I could not avoid it because she said she wanted to drive to Sherman to look for something. I had not known it prior to yesterday, and it was a total surprise to me. When I told Helen, she expressed great shock, and said that I was a traitor for "telling on her ". Of course I had not told anyone, but I was informed by the Area Alzheimer's Specialist of the state law that said if Helen were to be involved in an accident, even if it was not her fault, we could be sued, and our income would vanish overnight. So I will do all in my power to see that she goes where she wants as long as I or someone else drives. I feel for her because she thinks everyone wants to control her and/or take away her independence. Actually, driving her is an additional burden on me, but she doesn't see it that way. Knowing she has dementia and at the same time losing her driving privileges is a lot for her to handle right now. She needs time to deal with it. You asked if Celeste could help. She already has to a large extent. I can phone her anytime on her cell phone.

Celeste picked up Helen here and took her to her home last Tuesday and the next day took her to see the neurologist in Fort Worth. After the doctor's visit, Celeste returned Helen here the next day with instructions for Helen's meds which are rather complicated to say the least.

Each day is broken up into four parts -- morning, noon, evening, and bedtime, and each time period has requirements for particular meds. This alone is a rather time-consuming job. She doesn't argue with me about taking her meds, and I must keep up when to reorder them. She has at least ten each day, some being taken three times a day. . . .

Love, Charles

On June 25, 2009, Ellen wrote:

Dear Charles--and dear Judy too!

I've mentioned before, when Ken's sister Shirley was in the early stages of dementia, Ken & I were still making excuses for her: "She's eccentric; she has always been scattered and absent-minded, *etc.*" Near her 80th birthday when we called her she announced that since she was 80 she couldn't drive anymore. I explained that Ken still drove and he was 81. But no matter what we said it was as if she didn't hear us; she kept repeating she was 80 and couldn't drive anymore. I'm wondering now if there was

some kind of incident with her car, and maybe the authorities told her she must no longer drive. You know, like they've told you about Helen. [Ken was Ellen's husband who passed away.]

Long after that we learned that Shirley sometimes went out walking, looking for things in places where they wouldn't be found, like her car in someone's office. That's when Beth stepped in. Maybe Helen doesn't have the energy to wander, and your property is too large, but you might be on the lookout for that. Another things to look for: Shirley was always pretty good-natured. But there came a time when she became very ornery, later even psychotic & paranoid. The nurses took it in their stride, used to this, but we worried about it, about Shirley's obvious distress and fearing the nurses would become impatient.

Okay, so the nurses took it in their stride, but can you? Charles, this is going to be so tough! I don't think I could stand it. But I'll bet you hope to see this through yourself rather than drain your savings. It's a terrible choice. Lucky you haven't asked for my advice because I wouldn't have anything intelligent to say. . . .
Love, Ellen

On June 10, 2009, I wrote Ellen:

This afternoon I have an appointment with the area Alzheimer's specialist. I hope to gain important information to help me deal with what will ultimately develop. I hope to get some information concerning legal questions although I have dealt with a few of them already. But you know about legalities: there's always at least one more items to check out. I have a family attorney who will help in case his services are required. He is really an excellent attorney who has his client in mind when doing his job.

I really haven't anything much more in mind until I next email you. Last night Helen asked me when her husband would

return. She forgets so many things now. I have to write down things for her, but that doesn't always work. Anyway, I'm doing the best I can right now.
Love, Charles

The same day, Celeste emailed me:

Dr Lewis is unable to fill Mom's other meds and has recommended a Care Now facility, like a "Doc In the Box". An Urgent Care spot. I don't know what yours are called but it's like a local place you can go to that is a place to see a doctor if you don't have one. I am sorry I couldn't talk them out of one month of scripts. I am disappointed too. Did the PCP you got for her make her an appointment soon? How is everything going? I am almost afraid to ask. Love, Celeste

My answer to Celeste was:

Yes, we have an Urgent Care unit here, but we also have a family doctor, and both of us have a duel appointment on Monday at 3:20 PM. It was the earliest appointment I could get with our doctor. As far as Helen is concerned, she is accompanying me to see our doctor. I seriously doubt that an Urgent Care doctor will prescribe the Enalapril or the Methotrexate without having her medical records in front of him/her. I understand that, but it means that Helen won't have the Enalapril for weeks. She has been out for about two weeks before that. So I am doing the only thing I can legally do – make an appointment with our local family doctor. I think if I ask him he will write the scripts because I have never lied to him since I began seeing him more than 13 years ago. We'll have to see how that works out. The reason we are in this fix is because Helen would not let me drive her . . . to see Dr. Robinson to renew those prescriptions. My back is against the wall about all this. I am doing the best I can when trying to deal with the medical community.

This afternoon I spent nearly two hours with the Area Alzheimer's Specialist who gave me a lot of information. I can honestly say I have been oriented.

I found out how the state services work and what I can do to get Helen the maximum benefits. I still have much to learn, but I have taken a first step.

As I look back, Helen began showing symptoms of dementia about the time she began developing *prurigo nodularis*. If the ointment she is using is affecting her dementia, then I will have to ask Dr. Stevenson, the dermatologist, to find something else. But how in the world will I know if that is true? So I am going to let it ride because the ointment seems to be helping her to get better in that department.

She seems to be in a good mood today. I try to keep everything light. I merely suggest that it is time for her pills; she "seems" to be taking them okay now.

It's almost time for dinner, so I'll close. Thank you again for all your help. I wish I had good news.
Love, Dad

One subject that also dominated my thoughts was, Do I place her in a nursing home, and if so, when?

Celeste wrote, in part:

I love her and don't want to try to put her away until she's insensitive to it. That could be five or more years. Or one; you never know.

I responded . . .

Charles R. McCain Ph.D. & Celeste Barefield RN, BSN

I am really doing OK finding information about how to house Helen. I CAN use Medicaid. This week I have spent nearly two hours with the Area Counselor and Alzheimer's Caregiver Specialist about the legal, medical, and financial aspects of Helen's disease. I already have a letter from Dr. Lewis about her condition. I won't be able to afford the very "best" facilities, but I will be able to send her to a nice place. The Medicaid amount limit is adequate for a non-private facility. I would be responsible for the rest.

Now, the part which will be the glue that makes all this possible: Helen & I each have separate Wills (as suggested by our attorney). I must rethink all this ASAP and change all legal documents to reflect your involvement. I now believe that you should have Power of Attorney over Helen (now stay with me on this) and me if I should not be able to carry out the task of taking care of her. If it is necessary for you to do all that, it is a big job, believe me. I am not immune to Helen's disease although I am not aware of it in my family. I could die of a heart attack (which IS in my family) or die in an automobile accident, or in a host of different situations. I think you get the gist of what I am saying.

In addition, if Helen is mentally disabled, and I am either dead or not able to assist, you will be the person dealing with our estate. I also suggest that you consider Monica [Celeste's daughter] as your backup in case you are not able to carry out the functions. Eventually, you will have to make a Will anyway. Monica is a grown woman and should be able to help. She may as well get some experience with these matters because later in life she will likely make use of the experience. But that is up to you. I urge you not to involve anyone who is presently not in the family.

I'm sure I have given you much to think about. Take your time, but not too much time. I showed Helen a picture of us in 1982 at your grandmother Lola's house just across the field where we are now. She still doesn't accept that we are married, but I could have made a little headway there. Her denial of our marriage seems to come up late at night when she is tired. But each morning she gets up seemingly almost normal . . . another example of sun downing.

I am very tired now, so I am closing. I'm as close as your computer or your telephone. Hang in there!!

PART 8

Just One of the Guys

ONE OF THE most frustrating aspects of dealing with Helen was that she never did really say she believed we were married, but in the latter stages of her disease she didn't bring it up again. I saved a particular email to Cousin Ellen from June, 2009 which described the situation:

Dear Ellen:

. . . I spoke too soon about Helen's disease. Monday night she reverted to her old self and really dished it out. She thought I was just "one of the guys" and wanted me to leave again. She has several imaginary male "friends". When I wouldn't leave she called the Sheriff. I spoke with the officer on the phone and explained the situation. Of course he understood. After the call, Helen became enraged, telling me I was trying to control her. I know I can't control anyone and told her so. She then marched off to bed knowing that the game was over. But she will forget last night after the evening meal tonight. I have no earthly idea what will happen. She usually comes right off the wall with her assertions sometimes surprising me,

I have made an appointment with my family attorney to draw up new papers to assist me in this process. If she persists with her current behavior, I will have little choice but to move her into an institutional environment -- something I don't want to do. "Buckle your seat belts; it's going to be a bumpy ride." [A Bette Davis quote]

Celeste tried hard to settle Helen's problem with being married to me. In an email on June 16, 2009, she wrote:

Dear Dad:

When I called Mom, I told her that I remembered you two getting married and that I brought the wedding cake, and I described the cake, white with red roses and silver leaves. It said merry me or something and that it was close to Christmas 27 years ago. I "suggested" that since she was having memory problems that she let people like you and me who were not having problems help her remember things. I reminded her that Dr. Lewis wanted her to take Aricept to help her memory very day. She said she was. But she also told me that you were not the right Charles and that you were not married yet. I assured her that you were the same Charles and that's why you and she have the same last name because you are married and that she could look at both of your drivers licenses and see that.

I hope that did help and not hurt. Love, Celeste

PS The reason I wanted to come there was to introduce you in person, so to speak, and assure her that you are the right Charles.

The same day I answered her:

Dear Celeste:

I think we'd better stop trying to deal with her logically. Very late tonight (or early AM) she again got it in her head that I was not her husband. I tried to show her wedding photos and anything else that would prove my status. But she would not listen. She said she kicked out some other fellows, and it was my time to leave. I said a flat "no", so she called the city police. She handed me to the phone, and I spoke with the officer, explaining the situation. He understood. Anyway, the city cops have no authority out here -- it's the sheriff, but she doesn't realize that.

I think she has gone to bed now; it's 2 AM, so I think I'll do the same.

Please don't get upset again, I'll admit, she's a formidable, stubborn woman, but I'm determined to stick this out. Sunday and most of today were really pleasant around here until very late tonight. The fit hit the shan. I'm trying to ensure she takes her meds, and I think she has at least most of the meds the past two days. I don't know what the trigger is to set her off on this kind of tangent. I may never know.

I say there is still no reason for you to drive all the way up here and do what you said in your last email. I have an appointment with my family lawyer on Friday to go over all my legal documents and make any changes so Helen will be cared for if I am unable to do so. I have her power of attorney, so I have a number of chores to do with legal documents. I am asking you if you will be the executor or our estate when and if it becomes necessary? That means dealing with the financial aspects. Anyway, I will have to sit down with you and explain each document as soon as they are done. My Will won't change THAT much. Anyway the Will is very specific about the dispersal of the funds.

Well, it is very late, and I'm tired. Thanks for your support. Goodnight. It's after 2:30 AM now.
Love, Dad

Helen finally reached the county sheriff for the second time in June, 2009. The deputy who responded, had the authority to take her to the county hospital for observation in the event she had been physically abused. My family doctor visited her to ensure that she had not been harmed in any way. I was called that I could pick her up by Noon. I did. She looked very satisfied that I had been hassled because, after all, I was her "jailer". I took her home. Hardly a word was spoken in the car. She went right to her room. She said she didn't sleep very well in the hospital due to the noise in the hall and being awakened by nurses.

A couple of days later while Helen slept, I emailed Ellen about what had happened:

Dear Ellen:

Helen's behavior has leveled out since being sent to the hospital. For the most part, she seems to be happy. She still doesn't recognize me as her husband but does not complain. Last night she asked me to see if I could find her husband who seems to be "missing". I told her I would do it (I was lying). If one did not know her, she would seem as rational as any other adult until she mentions events that happened 30 years ago. Evidently some of the time she is still in the 1975-80 mode when she was at the end of her last marriage. They divorced, and he is dead, but she doesn't remember that. Anyway, that's why I don't have as much time for emails as I once did. I sometimes can do some things if she takes a nap in the afternoon. Her greatest problem is not being able to find something at which time I go over the house and find it where she last put it!

Gotta go now. I'm leaving for my appointment soon.
Love, Charles

In July Celeste offered to take Helen on a trip West (Texas, New Mexico, and Arizona). Helen jumped at the chance. I suspect Celeste did that to give me a break.

Later, I wrote Ellen:

Dear Ellen:

Helen will be back home tomorrow. And yes, I am "resting", something I really need. I nixed driving to Dallas because I would just get even more tired. So I am mostly staying home until tomorrow. Helen *is* a handful, but I am determined to do all I can. I have made a huge effort to make her life as pleasant as possible. I told her it was unlawful for her to drive because she has dementia

(I may have lied, but my attorney says if she has an accident that I am putting my entire finances in jeopardy if we are sued.) So she complains that she has lost that part of her independence. And I feel for her on that score. So life goes on.

Helen insists she does *not* have Alzheimer's, but Celeste says she does. The neurologist has not put it in writing yet. If he does, it will make my effort to begin to qualify Helen for Medicaid so she will have a good chance to get into a nice nursing home when the time comes. I just hope I have the "right stuff" to go the distance in this process. When trying to deal with her, I sometimes want to scream, but I don't because she cannot help what she is doing or saying.

Well, I need to fix something to eat, probably pizza from the freezer to the microwave.

Bye for now.

Love, Charles

A few days later Ellen wrote:

Dear Charles,

Guess Helen gets back today. You seem to have a good attitude toward her. You understand her condition, and that's the basis for your patience. I know you must become impatient sometimes -- you're not a saint -- but I believe you're going to handle this very well on the whole. But as I look at your road ahead, I'm wishing you all the fortitude and good will you'll need to see this through. Give yourself lots of breaks; you'll need them.

Love, Ellen

P.S. -- Interesting that Helen doesn't believe she has Alzheimer's. I can almost see how that would be; for some time at least a person still feels like herself. But I think when one begins to feel mixed up or struggling with something not understood she would feel irritated and frustrated.

PART 9

The Volcano is Rumbling

LATE JUNE, 2009 I emailed Celeste:

I hope your weekend was not very busy, at least less so than the one just before you came and picked up your Mom. We had a quiet weekend and enjoyed the lower temperatures. Today the temperature here didn't get much over 90.

Late last night Helen asked me if I would be sure and take care of the kitties. I told her that I surely would. She said she wouldn't be able to do that when she found a new place to live, something she can call her own. I just went along with it. Today she didn't say anything about it, so I didn't bring up the subject. I suspect she has already forgotten about it.

I took her to the dentist today because she had a gum problem; then we got a sandwich, picked up the prescription (antibiotic), and came on home.

Thursday I have another appointment with the family attorney. Helen has wanted a couple of changes, so I will see that that the new document reflects her wishes.

Have you managed to change the appointment with Dr. Lewis? If you do, please let me know. Helen doesn't like surprises. I need to be able to "remind" her often so she will be ready to see him again.

Well, time for the evening meal. Bye for now.

Love, Dad

Celeste and I exchanged several emails the last week of July, 2009. Here is a representative sample:

[July 22]

> Dear Celeste:
> Well, the meltdown came about 9 PM. She started by telling me (again) that I had to leave before her husband comes home. Again I told her I WAS home. She was relentless, following me all over the house ordering me out of the house. I DO know one thing -- I can't take this kind of verbal battering for much longer. I think she is my punishment for all the misdeeds of my life. I'm in a living hell right now. Something has to give.
> Bye for now.
> Love, DAD

Another e-mail:

> Dear Celeste:
> I had no idea that the disease would affect Helen as it has. Although I now know better; this is almost a comedy. She called my cell phone number I keep posted on the wall and left two messages. She thinks the man on the other side of the cell phone is her husband, not me. I'm saving those voicemail messages for you. It's a strange feeling --almost like I have a split personality, and I'm listening to someone talking to my alter ego. Earlier she threatened to call the police if I didn't leave. I believed her. If she continues this kind of behavior, none of the law enforcement agencies in this county will respond even if she really has an emergency.

From then on Helen only seemed to grasp reality at random times, mostly during the day. At night before she turned in she could be most difficult.

Painting with the Clouds

Late that month I wrote Celeste:

Dear Celeste:

The last couple of days have been *relatively* calm. At times she seemed to be her old self. Thursday night she again asked me to go to my home. Again, I told her "NO!" She said she would call the police if I didn't leave. This went on the usual way until I finally got rather irritated and got up close to her face and yelled that if she continued this childish behavior that I would have her committed to a place she would not like. Then I literally pushed her out of the computer room, shut the door, and locked it. I opened the door a few minutes later, and she had retreated into the South bedroom and shut the door. Friday morning she was a bit cool, but as the day wore on, she warmed up to me. That afternoon she asked me for a printout of my drivers license which I did for her. A few minutes later she asked me if I was the Charles McCain she married. I said "Yes." Today she has been for the most part her sweet old self. *But* I am aware that with Alzheimer's this could change instantly, so my antenna is up. She prepared a decent meal tonight (pork chops and rice). And she helped me clean up the kitchen at 10 PM. She is also taking her meds four times a day. Right now she is watching a rerun of "CSI Miami", a program she likes very much. After her bath, I will place Band-Aids on her skin wherever she wishes. I have one more email to send to cousin Ellen. She daily asks how Helen is doing. In vague ways, I tell her. Ellen and Cousin June are both real close and both know Helen. They are both interested in Helen's progress, and they both know she has Alzheimer's.

I am struggling to get all the legal documents separated and scanned into the computer. When you next visit, I will have copies of all her documents. If you come during a week day, I will take you to our bank and get you set up so you can get into the safety deposit box since I will put all the originals of our Wills

31

and other legal papers there. I will do that in the next few days. You will have power of attorney over either or both of us in the event I cannot function to handle routine business. Of course, Monica is your backup. I will try like hell to have everything in order when you visit. Whew!!

I hope your weekend is lighter than the last two. I hate to see you so tired. I hope you can convince your supervisor of the things you want in order to do a better job.

Helen said to tell you "hello." Don't worry needlessly about her. I don't think she will assassinate me in the middle of the night regardless of her disease.

I need to write one more email to Ellen, fix Helen's bandages, and go to bed. I'm tired.

Bye for now.

Love, DAD

In August, 2009, her paranoia became rampant. I wrote **Celeste:**

I was too tired to email you last night after the sheriff's deputy left. He was a sergeant and very experienced. I think rather quickly he saw what was happening. However, I furnished him with any I.D. he requested. He was most courteous to Helen and me. When she asked him to escort me out of the house and the property, he declined saying that all the evidence pointed to my residence here. Very softly he asked her to not push so hard. As he left he told me he would inform all the deputies about Helen and her inclination to call 911. He may even be able to place something on the police computer about her calling the cops. When she gets into that SUN DOWNING mode, there is no stopping her, so I imagine the cops will ignore any call she may make in the future with a complaint that a stranger is in HER house and won't leave. I hate that because she has cried "Wolf,

Wolf" twice before, and one of these days there may be a Wolf in the house.

As punishment, she has hidden the TV remote somewhere, thinking she is punishing me. That remote is the only one that will control the living room TV. More on that as it occurs.

I have no idea if she remembers her behavior last night. Last time she didn't remember some of it. This kind of behavior really disrupts my ability to take care of the house and property. Today the yard is to be mowed. I think some of the grass is about ten inches high. Tomorrow she has a dental appointment; I hope she agrees to go. Yesterday, she had her eyes examined for new glasses. We didn't have time for her to check out frames at Wal-Mart; I hope we have time for that tomorrow.

She awakened a while ago and came into the kitchen, but she didn't say anything to me. She did take her morning meds. I have to be "Johnny-on-the-spot" to ensure she gets her meds throughout the day even though the pill caddy tells her when the meds are due to be taken. I've a feeling that if I don't "remind" her, she won't remember to take them. That's one reason why I know she can't live alone. At the same time, I'm not sure I can physically & mentally tolerate her bad behavior for a very long time. When this happens, it exhausts me and interferes with my attempting to take care of her living here. I've made some inquiries about long-term care, but it is a slow process.

I must close because I have some bills to pay on-line.

Bye for now.

Love, Dad

Toward the end of 2009, I was becoming very weary mentally. Deep down I knew I could not sustain my role as caregiver indefinitely. My family doctor strongly advised me to place her in a nursing home where the people there are much better able to take care of her. He said that I would become a victim if I did not make that choice soon. He is an excellent physician, and I listened to him. Even with all the medications, she was not getting any easier to live with.

In August I wrote Celeste:

> I apologize for being a crybaby. I don't have anyone here to talk with. Living out here six miles from town has its disadvantages, and that is one of them. Thank you for the encouraging messages.
>
> Today I settled the bill from the hospital for her 24-hour stay last month. When she does these things, it drains our resources. I am looking into long-term-care insurance to "help" with the finances. I'm not sure she can get it, but I am going to try. I haven't applied for Medicaid; there are some financial requirements I must meet. The county Medicaid benefits counselor gave me a lot of information. I will be contacting him as soon as I get more information gathered.
>
> Today was as normal as one could ask. She went to bed about 10:15 PM, and she took all her meds as she usually does. She hasn't felt very good today. She says the allergy season is the real reason.
>
> I really don't know where her "mean" personality comes from. I have never abused her in any way since we have been married. I have tried to make life for her as easy as I could. If anything, I have spoiled her. She has never wanted for anything all these years as far as I know. But she sometimes acts as if we were at the poverty level and doesn't like to buy some things unless they come from her favorite store.
>
> That's it for today. She wants me to cancel her dental appointment for tomorrow because she doesn't feel well. I will call in the morning and try to do that.
>
> We are both looking forward to seeing you next week. In the meantime, stay cool.
> Love, Dad

On August 30, I wrote to Judy:

> **Helen is doing about as well as one can expect. She takes her many meds each day without a whimper. They seem to be helping her not to get any worse. But I know as time goes on that she *will* get worse, much worse. It is on my mind each day, but I have to move on so I can help her all I can *now*. Ninety-nine percent of the time she is easy-going. But that ONE percent is . . . , well, I won't go into that now. It is better explained in person. I am just taking all this a day at a time; I am not projecting any expectations into the future because it isn't too bright.**
>
> **I'm a bit tired now, so I think I'll close. I really appreciate your messages. I know you are on a close schedule.**
>
> **Take care.**
>
> **Love, Charles**

In September Celeste wrote:

> **Dear Dad:**
>
> **I am truly sorry if you have a rough time with her because I got her stirred up. She was being such a selfish pain, and I finally lost my temper with her. I just don't know how you can do it (stay sane) day after day with her. I don't do Alzheimer nursing for a very good reason. I need to be able to apply logic and education in my nursing and you just can't with Alzheimer's patients. She has also recaptured her ability to "push my buttons" since she started the Namenda. She knows how to turn a phrase to piss me off again. She had lost that ability for awhile there, but it is back. She always knew how to do that before she started this dementia, and now she is able to do it again. She made some smart remark about Michelle and me and our "so called relationship", while I was trying to seriously ask her not to disrespect you to me, and at some point in all that I lost it. I cracked. I am so sorry, to me**

that was akin to elderly abuse. Although, sometimes, I can't help but question, how much of her behavior is a put on, but I know my behavior was wrong, whether hers was or not. You can tell her that I apologize if you think she needs it. Hopefully, she will forget it before I see her again.

She started asking questions this time about Gramma Lola, after having seen her ghost recently. She wanted to know what was left to her and what was left to [her dead brother] Dennis. I told her half of the land was hers. She said that "they", meaning you, "told her that Dennis had gotten it all and none of it was hers" I told her that I was sure she misunderstood because you would never lie to her. I also told her in answer to her many questions that I would take care of everything and that I was helping you take care of her interests and that if need be I would retire there on the land. I would build a home there also so I could help. She was quick to tell me "no" on that one, that you and "the others" wouldn't approve and I would find it boring out there, *ad nauseam*. I think it would be a good idea to remove the temptation from Mom as she is still thinking she should "be allowed " to drive. If this is not an option, fine, but whatever you do . . . .keep me in the loop ! Love, Celeste

PART 10

Sundown Is Approaching Fast

THIS SEGMENT OF my report is not a summary. How does one summarize a human being's last days? Writing this account has dredged up some very sad times in my life. I decided to put these events in writing to honor my wife. There is no reason to "feel sorry" for anyone. Her disease made her difficult at times, but she became a relatively happy resident of a nursing home, especially the last 12 months of her 75 years.

Here, I am going to write about the last few months *before* she was admitted into a nursing home.

In November, 2009 Helen was still able to go with me to various places in the local economy. She was usually well-behaved. No one would have known of her problem without prior knowledge. On this subject, I wrote Celeste:

> Between both of us, Helen and I have four medical appointments through the 16th. I have one tomorrow; Helen & I have one with the dermatologist on the 9th; I have another with the "ear" doctor on the 13th; and I have a dental appointment on the 18th. So far we each have one in December: Helen sees Dr. Lewis on the 16th, and I have one with our family doctor on the 18th.
>
> Last night Helen again asked me to go to my home since it was getting late. I "reminded" her that I was her husband and would sleep in the house as I have been doing for more than 15 years since we arrived here. She said she was still confused who my husband was with all the guys coming in and out of the house [that wasn't

happening]. There was no argument; she accepted what I said and went on to bed. I have been encouraging her to retire a bit earlier to prevent the idea of "sun downing". This was a minor incident. She relented quickly, and that was that. I am hoping there won't be any more of those incidents. Yesterday she asked me if I had any children. I told her again what I tell her when she asks that question.

We went grocery shopping a few days ago. I now have to go with her up and down the isles because she will get things we don't need or have plenty of. One can look at our grocery store room at home to know which items we have extra supplies of and those which we don't!

I hope you are resting and enjoying your time off. Again, we look forward to seeing you no matter when you visit.

Take care.

Love, Dad

Celeste answered:

I know about the husband confusion; she did that with me too. Then she would agree that you were it. She can't always keep that in mind. It is hard not to seem superior when you remind her of things but try. That's when she gets that rebellious nature -- when she feels that she is being treated like a child or like she's nuts or inferior in some way. If what she wants more of is cheap, let her have it; if she wants too much at the grocery, if it is expensive, tell her she stocked up on it already and there's still quite a bit. Or one can ask, "Didn't I see a bunch of that this morning when I made the list...yes, we have that already! We can save money there."

She was quite acerbic when I tried to let her know something she said wasn't true. I gave up really and was worn out by the time

I left. I love her but I get really tired from trying to redirect her and find ways not to argue with her! Love, Celeste

Knowing that I was keeping a "diary" of sorts about Helen's dementia, cousin Ellen wrote in November:

Dear Charles,

Just wanted to say a couple of things more. I think this subject, your personal experience with an Alzheimer's wife, will make an interesting book. I'm not aware of how many other books have been written about the perspective of one person going through an up-close experience. I do think that if there aren't books of this sort, there should be. . . .

About Thanksgiving, 2009, Helen had fallen into a routine around the house that suited her. I tried to make her daily life as pleasant as possible, but I think I really spoiled her [Well, ten lashes of the cat-o'-nine-tails for me!] Late that month I wrote Celeste:

Just a note to tell you that I think Helen feels even better because she actually has been working on her sewing machine to make something for the kitties. She had me to take apart one of the wood houses that I had originally thought the kitties would sleep in. Wow, was I wrong! Neither cat liked their new house. For quite a while the houses sat on the porch unoccupied and unused. Finally Helen brought the smaller house in and used it as a foot stool. A few days ago she asked me to take it apart so she could reline the inside. I told her we should keep this quiet because the cops could get us for constructing a "cat house"! She didn't really appreciate my humor, but I tried. She is napping now.

I'm snacking on potato chips now and sipping on tea. I guess I've said my piece for today. I hope your weekend is easy. Bye for now
Love, Dad

The next day I sent Celeste another email:

Your Mom is okay today. She got up late in a dark mood, but by the time we had dinner, she had perked up considerably. I went to town to get her some yogurt and cereal. I had gotten some fried chicken yesterday from Kroger along with some stuffing, so she didn't have to cook. I told her she was barred from the kitchen and that I would put it down. I did. Then I put the dishes in the dishwasher and turned it on. She seemed happy with that arrangement.

It's late, so I bid you goodnight.
Love, Dad

Although Helen "seemed okay", she had her moments, quite a few as I recall. While on the trip "out West" with Celeste, Helen complained a lot about me and what I had not done. To her, these were legitimate complaints in her dementia state.

In an email in December, 2009, Celeste wrote:

Dad, she has only complained that you wouldn't wake up and confront the "drunken visitor" who came into your home and then got into your car for warmth .... Doctor Lewis was saying to me right in front of her that this was a hallucination, and she argued with him that it wasn't; he turned to me and said, "Is she safe in her home? Or is she hallucinating?" and I told him" she was hallucinating", then she was mad at me *and* him. She said "I just won't tell anybody then". Dr Lewis said "No, take a picture, call 911, wake up your husband"; she said "he wouldn't wake up"

etc.. She wants to go food shopping when you go; she claims to never go out unless it's an inconsequential trip. She wants her car, she cannot imagine why "one little fender bump 10 years ago would keep her from driving". . . good grief. I just try to explain, but of course I don't know anything as far as she is concerned. She says she can easily tell the difference between a hallucination and something real, and apparently I do not *ect* . . . *ect* . . . so not worth the talk.

I told her it is like a waking dream which is normal for her disease process and to stop trying to make me guilty for it. I can't help it if she has these things. I am not trying to make her feel bad. Love, Celeste

Only a few months passed before she was admitted to a nursing home. In January, 2010 her paranoia grew rapidly to the point that she was causing problems not only with me but also for others not to mention Celeste. There was another incident with the sheriff which led to the decision to place her in the care of others.

PART 11

Helen (Goff) McCain's Alzheimer's Story

by Celeste Barefield, RN, BSN
(Letters to family)

June 10, 2009. Well, I could not feel sadder or more weighed down to have to tell our family that Helen has Alzheimer's disease. She came into it this year in kind of a full blown way at the age of almost 71. You see, she was having chronic migraines for years and then many tiny bleeds on the brain showed up on the MRI and she had noticed some mild memory loss. She had to brow beat the Dr. into giving her Aricept to help with her memory. But that small town Neurologist just couldn't find the source or help with her migraine headaches, Charles, her husband, didn't think he was much of a doctor, so I decided to ask her if I could bring her to a Neurologist here in the Fort Worth area that might be more knowledgeable and help with the migraines. She finally agreed.

We began visits here, with Dr. Lewis. He came highly recommended by another Neurologist who I was familiar with but was booked up for months. He kept her on the Aricept, and she was doing a little better. She had less of the memory problems, they seemed so intermittent that I began to wonder if they were real at all. The migraines began to taper off too. Which I was glad of, but again, I still couldn't understand, unless maybe they were anxiety driven. Why out of the clear blue was this change happening? Well, if you let down your guard you will get sucker punched! Our previous visit with Dr. Lewis was January, (It was our 3rd and the 14th month of his care). At that meeting Helen refused to draw the circle for the clox test, so the nurse drew the circle and mom drew in a 12/9/3/6 correctly, but that was all she put in. The nurse and I exchanged glances, but I was in denial. I decided she was just being her bulldogged stubborn self. She refused my next visit and said that she couldn't explain why but that there were house guests. Then about a month ago I went to see her on Mother's day, and she was acting very strange, paranoid-delusional, talking about things like Charles stealing things from her, situations with people that she claimed had been there that had never been there (the imaginary guests).

She was unable to do simple things that she ought to be able to do (got lost for 3 hours and couldn't remember her own phone number or address). It was mystifying, but alarming. Charles and I had several telephone contacts and I moved her appointment up by several weeks so the doctor could see her sooner. It was last week, I had a difficult time getting her to attend; she developed a paranoid delusion that I had appeared out of nowhere without warning and was planning to take her someplace for crazy people. It took a lot to get her to my place. Fortunately I had taken the week off work. Monica, my daughter and greatest shoulder to cry on, reminded me by telephone when I called tearfully frustrated, that I was a nurse and that I could give her some of the meds that she was already supposed to be taking to calm her down, and tell her about the day at the spa I had planned for us, a pedicure and manicure etc....and to go eat crab together etc... and it all worked.

Well, Dr Lewis nailed it. She had stopped taking her Aricept and no one knew when, because she would not allow anyone to help her with the meds. He told her to take the meds every day and she agreed, but even today Charles tells me she won't allow him to help. He will not make her do it, he respects her dignity in this, and I feel it would be better if he could find a way to talk his way into it. But we cannot agree on this. Mean time, since the Aricept masked the beginning of the Alzheimer's we got it full force when she forgot to take the medicine and it was not refilled. I refilled it myself and got her back on it, but if she takes it or not is her decision. It is the decision of a lady who can't remember why she should and doesn't want to. Thanks to Karen, my sister, I read the book *Still Alice* by Lisa Genova, a Neurologist, about Alzheimer's told from the point of view of the victim of the disease. As all this was occurring in the last month. It has been a great help to me and I hope all of you will read it too. **Love, Celeste**

PS -- I will be glad to send anyone a copy of the book who would like one. I also will be glad to talk with anyone who wants to talk about it. But, she doesn't know she has Alzheimer's disease and is in denial (big time) and doesn't want to hear about it. Don't try to argue with her if she tells you something that is so odd you know it is wrong; just say something neutral and move on.

I THINK SHE would like to hear loving things and be remembered by everyone from time to time if you have time to write a note.

PART 12

"In Sickness and in Health"

THE PREVIOUS PART of the story was told to you from my own stand point as a daughter because I know it best. I can put it most easily into words or "prose" as Charles says. But I really do want to share with you what my adopted Dad is going through too. While I don't always agree with his approach, he has to decide ultimately what he can deal with, and I do know that.

He has remained constant in his love for Mom throughout and because of this and his love for Monica and me and his sacrificial help with Monica's college, I call him "Dad" and mean it. He is a war hero, some people don't know it but he was a war photographer and got injured. He was a college professor for over 33 years. He's been Mom's husband for over 30 years. All commendable feats!

"In sickness and in health" has a whole new meaning when you are speaking of being married to Helen. She suffered from migraine headaches for 11 years, previous to arriving at Alzheimer's disease at a full grown moderate stage. Dad has been writing me letters about her allergies and memory lapses and migraines for years. I have been trying to help, but really what could I do from 2 hours away? He is living with her day after day after day. Sometimes I can't find the time to get the drive in for months…well let's face it, Mom and I never really got along all that well. I really have little patience with people who are "sick" all the time. I was probably too judgmental of her (as a nurse) and felt that she was faking all of her millions of allergies and migraines. I never could have handled her on a consistent daily basis as Charles has. Does that mean I don't love her? No, but I'd never marry her! Dad does love her! She asks him who he is twice a day and shakes her head as if she doesn't believe the answer, and hears things in the middle of the night which he faithfully investigates for her, knowing it's nothing. He's had the house checked for gasses, little bugs with gray wings, and repainted (for non existent mold). You name it he has done it to please this person who might not remember the demand so defiantly made as if he'd never done anything for her before. She thanklessly accuses him of theft of the very things he's given her, her wedding rings, the large ruby ring she lost, *and* the one he bought to replace that one. The rubies turned up, but so far we haven't been able to find the wedding ring or the ring I got her for Mother's day.

Since she got the skin disease called *Prurigo Nodularis*, he's had to deal with her intense itching 24/7. One problem with that disease is, it can last *for years*, and the people who have it are often convinced that it is caused by parasites, even when it is scientifically proven it is not. Well Dad has had to watch as the woman he loves tries to catch these creatures, listen while she discusses them at length and bandage the sores as she scratches and dissects them bloody time and time again. Meanwhile, trying to get them covered with an ointment twice daily and get Mom to take her pills to help with the itching. This is patience I am not able to produce, and certainly not maintain day after day. I thank God for Dad; his love for her has made all the difference in her life and in mine. What ever needs to be done to help, I am here, and I hope if any of our family has any way they can help him, they will certainly offer. **Celeste**

The little girl cried, "Wolf, Wolf"

WELL, FROM OUR perspective, Helen's Alzheimer's has been an unceasing battle of the egg shell walk verses the scramble to fix whatever happens when the egg shells crack! Helen has run away once, gotten lost several times and called the police twice so far. The small town police are now on to her and probably don't know how to respond when she calls anymore. Should there be a real emergency I wonder if they will really come. See, she cannot re-member Charles and is sure he is one of several men, all who go by the name Charles and claim to be married to her, none of which is actually Charles in her mind who are in her home for some unknown reason and are apparently drawn there by the computer! Go ahead and try to explain it all to her. I have, multiple times in multiple ways. Look at these pictures of your wedding day, remember? Hey I brought the cake, trust me *I* remember! But, oh no, that only lasts a few seconds and then her paranoia sets back in and she starts back down the same old beaten path.

You can't follow a train of logic that has gone off the track! Poor Charles, after 27 years, she calls the cops to try to get him kicked out of his own home; she told him to get out many, many more times than she finally called 911. She tells him she is ready to go to bed now and it is time for him to leave! He says no and the fight is on. What would you do? PUNT!

Charles has been long suffering, but face it he's 7 or 8 years older than she is and working to keep his health up. How much of this can one man stand? How much can I do? Not much. I try to be supportive, I go there ev-ery 2 weeks to give him a break, I take her to my place to let him have total freedom, or I take her to the neurologist, who she doesn't trust because he told her she has Alzheimer's. I take her to get a pedicure, manicure, hair cut and style. Just to give her a change of scene. We go do shopping therapy at Goodwill (her favorite store). But I have to tell myself this isn't really much help, Alzheimer's is incurable, it's degenerative and worse…it's terminal. I know in my nurse's heart that it's normal to feel ambiguity where the illness of family members are concerned. I wish it would go away or that it would hurry up and get past this part (when the next parts are inability to talk, walk, eat and eventually death)…then I wonder if I am a monster. Then I know again, this is normal. I am just a normal caregiver going through the normal stuff.

In a detached medical way I can see that to be involved in an Alzheimer's case of multiple personalities is interesting stuff. But in a personal way I can see where that really sucks donkey snot too. One minute you are dealing with a relatively sane, forgetful, thoughtful person who is appalled that she is not helping to support herself in any meaningful way. Then the next, she is telling you with a nasty sneer on her face that slitting someone's throat might be the quickest way to solve a problem! Her voice coming from a deeper scarier place, complete with demonic chuckle that sounds as if she'd had some experience with just that very event. Only seconds later to be gone without even a whiff of brimstone to remind you that the conversation ever took place. If you ask a leading question to try to invoke it again, it is gone, forgotten, swirled away into the black hole of the Alzheimer memory. It may or may not ever show its ugly unpredictable face again. Some scientific medical person might find that fascinating, I find it exhausting. I am sure that Charles, who is with her every day, finds it beyond punishment for all his sins. I wonder how anyone gets through this in one mental piece when the sick person is not the passive quiet type.

Helen has never been what you would call passive or the quiet type. I'd say that her 4 marriages would attest to the fact that she generally got what she wanted or needed, or she moved on. Charles made life tolerable for her for the last 27 years. Many thought that was amazing and saluted that it was possible.

Painting with the Clouds

We didn't know why or care how. But I know how now. He loved her enough to be self sacrificing and long suffering. That's what it would take. Not just anybody would do that.

And now this. There is a certain sound to his voice sometimes as we talk that hints to the days of better times when he says, "She's in personality #4 today; it's almost like the lady I met and married" I know he loves that lady. It's tough to get to be around #4 though. You have to hang around. One to three are the more common personalities to see. When you see that mean one though look out! It is by far the most dangerous and the cleverest. She even threatens to burn the house down if she doesn't get her way when she's in that personality. I believe she's dangerous to him and herself. Her main personality thinks people come in and steal from her. She invents people who come in, mostly they are friends and family of the Charles imposters...you know, the ones that look, act and sound just like him but aren't him? Well those bastards are all thieves and they steal stuff and wait until no one is looking and put the things back sometimes just to screw you up and make you look crazy so no one will believe you. Of course she just told you that story yesterday in full and may tell you that story again in 5 minutes too. If you tell her she already told you she says, "When did you tell me that?" and you say "No, Mother, you told me." She says, " I just did," and you say," Well of course you did", "Who's on first?" and give up. When she starts on him not being her husband I just change the subject now.

Sometimes when the mean one shows up she will say mean things to me, me! She and I have history now. I should have had her burnt, crushed fine, and spread out to blow away in the wind by assassins a long time past if you know what I mean. But here I am taking care of her like the dutiful daughter that I am trying to be. I figure I will be a better person because of it. And truthfully, I know she can never change the kind of person she was or is now. So, I guess I have been forced by my logic to move along. But, man it hurts when I see her being mean to Charles and when she is mean to me. When she is mean to me, I have to retreat to my nurse mode and mentally write nursing notes, like this:

"Patient is confused; poor historian, alert times person only; family dynamics strained due to patient's verbal combativeness; patient reoriented to location and time; medications given on time. Patient well nourished, appetite good although sense of smell appears to be lost, strong food tastes are preferred."

"Patient is overweight at 218# and 5'4", sob, ambulatory for moderated distances. Tires easily due to weight, and sob, no oxygen in use at this time. Patient has some pitting edema around the ankles, thought to be caused by increased sodium level due to excessive intake of diet root beer. Patient drinks about a 2 liter bottle daily. And eats a great deal of sweets, including a pint or two of ice cream daily. Patient is not diabetic."

Then a good nurse might continue; "Patient has Pruritis Nodularis, a skin disease primarily evidenced by itchy bumps that are easily scratched open and very slow to heal over approximately every square ½-1 inch of her body except her scalp, her palms and the plantar surfaces of her feet. Since she picks the open areas and the healing scabbed bumps repeatedly due to her dementia, the spots either become infected or heal very slowly and scar badly. Patient is unable to remember not to touch the spots, therefore the medications for the itching such as capsaicin cannot be used because of the danger to the patient of getting the oils of the hot peppers in the mucous membranes of the eyes, nose and mouth."

Notes such as these keep me neutral so that I can get out of my personal self and not react to the pain it causes when I feel hurt inside me. Charles has no medical training. I wonder what he does to deflect pain inside? **Love, Celeste**

Dementia *vs.* Knowing exactly What You Are Missing! Or: Sex, Drugs and Zen

ADDING THE NAMENDA to the Aricept has helped, but not enough. You can't stop this runaway train with a cow and a wall of hay; just slow it down twice a day. I take her to the doctor again soon, his reaction to all this will be; "You are doing fine. See you in 2, 4 or 6 months".

She keeps asking (in her more lucid moments) if there isn't some surgery, some medication or some retraining of her memory that could be done to help her get "back to normal". I have to keep saying, there is always hope that something will become available soon. The other thing she has asked twice now is "Am I going to lose my memories and my mind completely?" I cannot bring myself to be 100% honest about what all she is going to lose. How she could have forgotten what Alzheimer's disease really does to people I don't know, but there it is. She has always considered herself to be an intellectual. Truthfully, all the books she's read would fill a small library. How can I hurt her that much just because she has a lucid moment? Instead I told her it will be much like living every moment for today and today only, no fears for future needs or hassles and no worries of the past ever catching up to you! Every moment will be pure, without preconceived notions of whether or not you should or shouldn't and no one will place blame or accept it. She rather liked that. It did have a sort of Zen sound to it.

She broke through, one of her personalities understood for a time that Charles is the only one there at her home! Although she admitted outright she cannot find any memory of marrying him 27 years ago. She was mortified that she had treated him so badly and admitted that she never even gave a thought to the idea that someone was supporting her. She's never worked outside the home full time in her life, she has always had someone doing that; it is the natural way of things in her generation. She told me no one would hire her now except the owners of the place she's living in now.… Good grief off we went again.

The Namenda plus the Aricept has caused some thoughtful even deeply reminiscent times. She questions deeply then falls into denial at the truth while saying repeatedly that she's sure I would never lie to her. After all, what have I to gain by it? I expect the mean personality to forget the age difference between me and all those imposter Charleses and decide that we are all plotting to get her locked up so I can take her very old home (giving up my own $90,000 home I presume) and live a life of paradise in a run down small town that is a bedroom community for a failing midsize city.

Seriously, if paranoia wasn't a typical symptom of these early stages of the "walkie-talkie" Alzheimer patient; I would be like Charles and get upset. He gets so upset because she tries to kick him out ever so often and then she lets the mean personality take over and it's the really clever one. That, my friends is scary. Fortunately, if we make it through the night, the sweet personality rallies the next day and she's OK again for days or even weeks. Sometimes the Namenda makes her realize the things she is missing but doesn't help her with her natural "gatekeeper" which is lost completely where I am concerned apparently. What's a gatekeeper?

A Gatekeeper is what prevents us from saying inappropriate things at the wrong times in the wrong places. Everyone has them, except people that have Alzheimer's disease. For example: I took her out to a local bar and grill for lunch the other day; it's a small place, in the booming small town I live near. It is really a biker hang out named after an amphibian. The ambiance is American Macho with checkered tablecloths spread on wooden picnic tables or old fashioned booths. They have fans set up to blow on you and a big screen TV to watch whatever sports are on. You can enjoy the jazz piped over the speakers while you eat or if you are feeling outdoorsy, you can sit outside at wooden picnic tables and smoke, drink beer, listen to good music, and the bikers cussing and laughing while you eat. The food is excellent! I was sitting across from her in a little booth with my back to the two working types in the booth behind us. We were the only four people there at 2 pm, when she suddenly said in a moderately quiet voice "I really like sex. I need sex and you can tell Dad that!" I answered in a low voice, "Mom, what if you think it's not him, I wouldn't want you to try to hurt him, or feel like you were being raped or anything". She answered matter of factly, " I wouldn't care if it was one of the 'others' ", I hedged carefully knowing more than she can remember, "Well you know since the prostate cancer…", forgetting that she might not "get" a pregnant pause…to which she quickly and quite loudly replied, "Well, teach him how to use a vibrator! I can't do it myself and I need sex!" The two guys behind us picked up their food and moved to the table farthest away from us. I was mortified. Then I nearly died from trying not to laugh! No gatekeepers left!

Needless to say I did pass on this important information to Dad as a funny story and let him run with it in his own way; I hope she doesn't share the story of how it all turned out with me in another public place! **Love, Celeste**

Drugs: Restoration or Revivification; You can never go back!

WELL, THE NAMENDA has been working; she has been remembering more and has recovered some of her abilities to perform kitchen tasks such as simple cooking and cleaning. She at times even remembers her husband long enough to decide she wishes she'd married someone else. She actually told me she felt sad that I told her there was only one man (her husband) and not an entire group of suitors, she had fallen in love with one of them, he was taller, younger, slimmer and had impeccable manners, and she wanted me to know that if she got married she would have been leaving, but now she had no hope of that. Her husband has been wonderful and long suffering with her. Certainly, he has been more so than I have. To me this was disrespectful to him, in such a way that I could not stand it, and became so offended for him, I began taking my anger and frustration out on her through my driving. I drove fast and hard as only I can do with my sports car, knowing my capabilities, I know I scared her. She made one final mistake in all this when she referred to my relationship with the woman I love as a "so called relationship". I became so enraged at her button pushing, I actually yelled at her, to stop being such a selfish B***CH and felt guilty for showing my ass for weeks afterward. I know this is normal and all caregivers fall into this frustration sooner or later. With my head I know it, but with my heart I couldn't believe I'd done it, and me a nurse. But see, the Namenda has helped her remember how to be a selfish B***CH, which she has been to me all her life. Did I mention that we were not always on the best of terms, my mother and I? Well I almost liked her when she forgot how to push my buttons, with her smarmy, snide remarks about my hair color, makeup or clothing choices. Now I am rethinking how I can help him and spend time with her without wanting to crack her over the head with a bat! Just like the old days but not really…see she is still deteriorating underneath. I saw her reading the paper the last few days she spent with me, she's not actually reading it. She's scanning it for familiar words and pictures. It takes her literally hours to "look" at the news paper. Yet, she craves it daily and she will even say, "It doesn't matter what day it's from, or which paper" which is not like her at all! So while some things are obviously improved, the brain destruction goes on. I saw her two weeks after this, and while I know she remembers the angry scene, the very first thing she said to me as we got into my sports car to go shopping at her favorite store, *Goodwill*, "I wish you'd never told me that there's only one man". Truly, you can never go back. **Love, Celeste**

PART 16

Don't worry, be happy!
Life goes on!
With or without her
actually being ALL there!

WELL, I CALLED Charles to let him know about my vacation 11 days without the phone, patients, or bosses to stress me out, just the little woman, bills, my mother and home! Ha. Well mom answered the phone in her soft, "I am just the same Mom as I always was" sounding voice, and then proceeded to tell me about all those guys that come around and eat and then just go away, but she'd let Charles know I needed to talk to him if she ever saw him again. She tells me she's bored and that she's ruined a meal by over seasoning and over cooking it. I am not surprised. I noticed last time I was there that she cooks every thing on high, and can't remember how to work anything electronic. So, I asked if one of those guys was there, and she said, "Yes, did I want to talk to him? Good Grief! Yes, of course I did. She takes the phone to him (Charles, of course) and says "my daughter" as if we had never met. Lordy, Lordy, some days I cannot take it! I wish I could turn back the hands of time to…what? The mom I didn't get along with? I don't know, I am ambivalent about it. I wish she wasn't losing her mind and at the same time, I wish if she found it she would be a sweeter, less selfish, less egotistical, less demanding, lady. But that would never happen so … oh well.

She always remembers to ask about my partner Michelle, and I tell her she is fine and working. Since several years ago Michelle cannot be around my mother because my mother gave her a "look" when she was in the Evil Personality and deliberately (or so Michelle thinks) walked in on us one morning while she was getting ready for work. Michelle thinks it was deliberate because I had explained carefully to Mom the day before that Michelle is a very private lady, and that mother should not enter my bedroom, as she was in the habit of doing, until everyone was awake and out of the room. So, what was the first thing she did at the crack of 7am in the morning? Mom gets up and walks straight into my room and just stands there looking at us, as we stare frozenly back at her in our under clothing in various states of getting ready for the day. It wasn't until Michelle covered her front (she was wearing a brassiere) that the whole tableau snapped back into real time and I asked Mom if she'd give us a while. I did not see the "look" but I am told it would kill! I have to say it was 7am, and my mother is not one to rise before 12 on most days of her entire life. Heck, I can remember having to sign her name to my school notes if we forgot them because in her sleep states she could sign anything! She once signed "Mrs. Sam Houston"! I actually got where I could sign her lovely handwriting as well as she could…I could never write anything else that pretty, but I could sign "Mrs. R.D. Jones". Now her handwriting has a childish look to it, almost like she just learned how to write in script and her spelling is very poor. She has read more books than most small town libraries have in the adult collections, but she takes all day to read the paper now, and she doesn't even really care what day it's from, or for that matter what city it's from. I think she just looks at the pictures and reads the captions over and over trying to remember what she reads. It's sad, monumentally sad. Charles noted recently that in the newspaper obits was one that told of someone's 20 year long fight with Alzheimer's disease! He sounded panicked; I told him that at the rate she is progressing she might not have that long. I think his fear is that he will not outlive her and someone will have to take care of her and him, ME! But, I assured him that I can handle what ever pops up. He says financially he cannot afford to put her in a nursing home at about $4000.00 a month unless he dies first! Then his insurance money will pay for her care. I told him again not to worry. I will find a way no matter what happens. I know I will because I always have. I survived incest, rape, alcoholism, abandonment,

PTSD and now this. I have no fears anymore. I can make it through and will manage whatever pops up.

Have you ever noticed that no matter what you worry about you always get past it and you manage to survive it, whether it worked out or it didn't? Yet here you are, reading a book. That's because life goes on. Life really does just keep on keeping on.

Rest or Focus Challenged?

I HAVE AVOIDED writing about my mother for so long due to the fact that I have not seen her for a while. I had to have surgery and my life took a front seat for a while using up all of the time I had for extra time off. Now I will be visiting without time off so the driving will have to be out of my energy reserves. My job continues to be difficult and so many other thing are chiming in to keep me from focusing constantly on Mom and the problems there that I have had a good long rest. If rest is what it would be called? Perhaps the truth is my focus has been challenged in other areas.

However Dad has sent me a wonderful news article by Jonathan Rauch first published in the *Atlantic Magazine* © 2010 that is called "Letting Go Of My Father". I sense he is trying to tell me it is too much for him and that he wants to be able to commit her right away. I haven't had the heart to tell him what the true eventualities are for Alzheimer's disease. I can't tell him that she is far from the end stages and that she is far from being able to be kept anywhere she doesn't want to be at this point. She will cause so much trouble at this point she will get herself barred from every place out there. He sees her as almost unbearable as do I, but I know, in the real world she has a long way to go before it comes to commitment. She is still walking and talking and able to pretty much talk her way out of anything she wants to. She can still be a vixen (read that as a dirty word) of a woman any time she wants to.

I would love to see her in an assisted living for Alzheimer's patients and feel she would be safe there, but I know her too well. She'd wait until she had the opportunity and out she'd go and she'd find herself killed by someone, or become lost and die of the elements in no time. I feel the only way that will happen is to wait until the disease is advanced to the point that she is unable to speak a single word that makes sense or even until she can no longer walk.

He may not understand the physical problems that will descend on her about that time. I have not been able to bring myself to tell him. He is an intelligent man who is computer savvy and he can look it up in the right places, but will he? I don't think he will. I think he thinks that everyone is different and that the disease will be just the loss of her memory. How can I tell him that it could go on for 10 more years, and that in the last 10 she will forget how to swallow, how to know when to pee, or poop, how to walk, how to feed herself or wash her own face. I gave him a book to read but he told me it was too sad to read and I think he never read it. A great one called *"Still Alice"*.

I have often hoped this was just her faking it for attention, and I hoped that a real specialist would uncover the truth. But the neurologist didn't think so. I just have such a hard time with the fact that the first thing she forgot in its entirety was her marriage to her current husband. She claims she cannot remember her marriage to him at all. That was 27 years ago. Yet she claims to remember my daughter who is only 26 years old. She remembers my brother and me who are both older than this marriage. But has all the other marriages fuzzed out. This makes me wonder. But other things make me surer of it. She will forget we are coming to visit and get mad because she wasn't warned and isn't ready, she takes 2 hours to pack one 3 day suitcase; she can't remember to take her pills; and she can't cook anymore at all, things like that.

I have to admit, Mom and I have never been the closest of family members, but I don't want her to be dying of Alzheimer's. Old age is bad enough of a punishment for her. **Celeste**

Multiple personalities and they ALL have Alzheimer's

WELL HERE IT is summer in Texas again and HOT! Like 97 degrees with greater than 50% humidity. Helen has run away again, and is immured in a behavioral center that is related to the hospital in the next small city over. I was just in town visiting, and had spent time trying to calm her down again about her husband selling her car. She was just not safe with it, and he sold it to save money. She can't remember he is her husband and doesn't care that he spends their money on her to care for her. She is still in denial after five years; she certainly doesn't add much good to the mix at this point and is making him miserable hounding him constantly about stealing her car and trapping her against her will. So after I left she got meaner and meaner, and the mercenary personality called the sheriff and reported that someone had stolen her car and was trying to kill her. She got out the door while Dad wasn't looking and went out in the heat, in the middle of the day to stand outside near the gate (did I say in the 97 degree heat?) waiting for the sheriff. Poor Dad finally discovers she has absconded again and gets in his car to go find her and get her out of the horrible heat. He discovers the Sheriff at the end of the drive with mom in the back seat. So, the final deal is that the sheriff signed her into the behavioral center after a checkup at the hospital. The rest has been looking through her things to find the medicine she hid, clothes she has requested, and her jewelry to put into the safety deposit box. We talked to an eldercare lawyer and OMG that's expensive! Try $7,000.00. But well worth the cost He really did know what he was talking about. Dad found a nursing home with a locked unit for Mom. But now we have to actually get her into the home without her killing us or anyone else!

Digging through mom's things to figure out what to do with it all. There is stashed food. Ninety pairs of earrings, and 20 or more bracelets. She has hidden the real jewelry and I don't know where yet. About 20 pairs of shoes. A walk in closet packed tight with shirts and pants, and a rack full of shirts and pants. Charles tells me there are more bags of clothing in the shed. I have gone through boxes and boxes of junk. Buttons, clips, snaps, bobby pins, safety pins broken things, pieces of things I can't decipher, and magazines in the hundreds. Many notebooks with notes to herself, me or Charles. Most with only a few pages used at the front or back. Some of the notebooks are perfect examples of how her mind has gone downhill. The ones she dated 2-5 years ago, her handwriting was prettier and there were less spelling errors. She noticed the errors and wrote of them. She wrote of her hallucinations. She wrote about her demands. She wrote about her delusions. She even wrote about her political thoughts when she had some clear enough to put on paper.

Her main political thought was that Republicans are mean people. We need to stop participating in the wars these mean republicans keep starting. That of course, included me, naturally. But since I was young (in my 50's) I could not possibly know anything, so I was just a stupid Republican person (when it came to knowing anything at all about the real world) rather than a mean one. This was her normal self talking. When she used to get into political arguments she came spitting acid, cruel and nasty. That was the mercenary. She can't hold onto the political thoughts long enough to do that successfully now.

Well, I found only one of her 3 ruby rings. The other two are god knows where. I have been trying to locate anything of value to put in the security box at the bank. I have put my hand into pockets, shook out shoes and purses, gone though innumerable boxes of crap and so far nothing. She told me "good!" when I told her I couldn't find the jewelry she asked me to lock up for her. I said, "GOOD!? Why do you say that?" And she said, "Oh I mean it is not important now. I need to get out of this place." She has been in the locked unit now for 10 days and will not stop telling Dad that she will bust out. She has told him she will break out or will bang her head on the wall until she dies if she has to. I have told him she is trying to fool him. She also asks him to take her shopping for a few little things or an ice cream or some little something every time he visits. But, so far he is on to her. I can remember the last time she talked him into giving her the keys though. He still loves her, and she can still manipulate him. My step sister, the product of another marriage entirely, has been e-mailing with Dad and me about Mom. They had a tempestuous relationship. The fact that Mom only remembers my step sister Karen "sort of" is amazing. She HATED Karen for a long time! She felt that Karen trapped her when she took her car and wrecked it. Mom could have walked the one block to see her three best friends, but she always thought of herself as "trapped" without a car. She was mean to Karen and never really forgave her even though Karen worked off the debt. She could have had a car anytime; she was not willing to work to have it. She worked at a pet store for a very short period of time and then just stopped. She was always too "nervous" to work. She and several friends who drank, read, and had the kids to do everything for them were the intellectuals. It was the drink alcohol, claim nervousness, take Valium and let the village raise the kids generation. That tail end of *The Silent Generation*, the parents of *The Baby Boomers*, us. Most of the older daughters got pregnant. Of her and three girlfriends, we had six pregnant out of wedlock teen daughters! Sad isn't it. My generation didn't do a whole lot better. But we are the Yuppies now! Mom's memory is lost back to 1968-69 now I guess. **Love, Celeste**

Helen's final chapter?
A very important message
in the Clouds?

Mom has been sick with Alzheimer's disease for at least nine years that we knew of. She began acting "different" at least that long ago. She had managed to get a doctor to prescribe Aricept for her "memory" and we didn't know she was having dementia until it got strong enough to make her forget to get her refills. Suddenly my mom was this "seemingly crazy" person. She went from zero to sixty over night. This was the hardest thing. I always said that she'd read enough books in her lifetime to fill a small local library. She was an intellectual and proud of her reasoning capabilities. Then she started to have paranoia and aggressiveness. She began to think her husband of nearly thirty years was a multitude of strangers who looked and acted like her husband but were not him. Every time he left the house he returned as another stranger. She thought it was a group of people she worked for as a cook and housekeeper. At one point she thought he was trying to kill her.

On the other hand he was her protector when she heard people outside in the night or saw homeless drunks in her bedroom that covered their eyes when they saw her. Once she saw a tiny black demon run under her dresser (on two legs). She became convinced that she has parasites in her skin and collected bits of skin by taping them to paper saying that these things were proof that her itching was parasitic. She actually thought she saw eyes on the spots she scratched and picked at until she bled. One very hot Texas day she left the home unnoticed and walked across a busy country road and asked the people there to call the police because a man claiming to be her husband was trying to kill her. She refused her medicines, paranoid that they were something that was part of a plot to kill her. Mom felt that everyone else was wrong about reality; it wasn't her at all. It was all of us.

When she got lost in the car for several hours, we took away the keys. We sold the car, and that was a biggie. All hell broke loose and finally we ended up putting her in a behavioral hospital. We tried everything to help, but it was not just an illness, it was a degenerative brain *disease*. There was no cure and little to help. She had to live in a locked unit where she could not wander and hurt herself or anyone else in her paranoia. That was the hardest thing (I say that a lot). Watching her degenerate from a lively, talented, artistic person into a sort of automaton; that was it, the hardest thing. She paced up and down the halls and talked in a suspicious tone about everyone there. She decided it was some sort of school she'd been sent to and most of the women staff were actually men. She thought the other people were unable to communicate well, so when they talked together, (none of them saying one single intelligible word), that they were all co-conspirators against the machine. Later on she forgot to worry about this. For Mom, eventually, it was like waking up in a new and confusing world every day. She always said the food was good, and that she was treated well. Yes and no answers really. I always wondered how she knew, since she couldn't remember anything current for more than a few seconds. She had started to dissect her meals into "packages" wrapped in napkins or anything she could find, and offering them to the others there at the nursing home. This was sort of humorous as she used to go around helping herself from the other resident's plates as though at a buffet before. The other residents and she often traded things, things we had given her. She gave away and received jewelry, stuff animals, art work and dolls...she was one of them now. My mother was gone, but Dad and I tried to see that she had everything she needed, knowing all along that someday, before we knew it, she'd pass away.

Well it finally happened. She just stopped eating and drinking. She had been going along slower and slower for the last few weeks. Mom was losing weight, a lot of it. She had lost who I was a long time ago. She remembered to pretend she knew whenever I asked, and if I said, " What's my name Mama" she'd laugh and tell me something totally in gibberish. I never learned gibberish, I just went by her mood, and her face looked like she really didn't recognize me and was not too sure I was OK.

The doctors at the hospital said that they might be able to re-hydrate her and get her kidneys going again, but as long as she wasn't on tube feedings for the rest of her life it wouldn't help. She definitely did not want that. Dad was certain of that, she'd made her wishes known. "No heroic measures".

So she rested away in a very peaceful manner. I was at her side, holding her hand. There was a tiny 20 second seizure; I prayed the Lord's Prayer and sang to her quietly. I had been praying that Grandma Lola and Grandma Jewel would come to mama and help her find her way. I told her to look towards the light. She was gone just minutes later. Comfortingly, her arms stretched out and then gently crossed her chest as if in a quiet hug, just as she left me. Now she was free of her wounded body and broken mind. It was as she would have wanted it to be.

On the highway on my way home days after the funeral, I clearly saw the first four letters of my name in the clouds right in the middle of my windshield. She was an artist; I thought to myself, she's painting with the clouds and wanted to prove to me she was well and like the Bible says, "We will be as He is". Only God can paint the sky, right? No, now she can too. If she had written my entire name in the clouds a bunch of people would have noticed, perhaps even photographed it, as it was, it was a message (a gift) just for me. She said, "I'm fine and look what I can do"! I also came face to face with a hummingbird where there were no feeders and few flowers as well. It looked me over and zipped away apparently satisfied. It is also written God takes care of the birds, and now she does too. Theologically this presents a whole new way of thinking.

She is in heaven (whatever you think that is) and has the powers or characteristics of God. She had studied all the church history and was active in her church before Alzheimer's came along in her life. She was fascinated by angels and had many books of paintings of angels. She had last rites as well. What does all this mean to me? She transformed back into God. She became part of what or who God is again. This is a tremendous comfort to me. If your loved one has died, trust in the thought it is a transformation, not the end. Look for signs in nature that your loved one is just fine. I know this for a fact now. I am so grateful to know this as I too have had the migraines and fear that I will be an Alzheimer's patient someday too.

The patient with Alzheimer's brain was once described to me as a round hall with many doors, behind which are the realities of millions of sets of the realities of lived memories; this hall spins around and periodically stops at a door which opens and that reality is now present in all it's glory to be lived again (however confusing it might be). Since the Alzheimer's patient is having constant degenerative brain damage, the most recent memories are unreachable, but the older ones are still intact. This may be why these people cannot be convinced at any given time that their mother was not "just here", or "waiting to take you home" because that was 60 years ago and she's dead now. The reality "feels" so real because it includes all the recorded info of that moment. Naturally confusion, paranoia and sometimes aggressive anger is produced by this mind, leaving the patient with no one to turn to for help. They are fortunate if they can recognize a friendly face and feel secure for the visit, no matter what the brain is doing.

I used to say that you can't find logic to explain reality to Alzheimer's patients because the logic train has jumped the track. They do not get to choose the destination of the spinning hall of doors but are subject to the reality wherever it stops. Our brains are absolutely filled with the characteristics of this very moment. We are cataloging the sounds, feelings, situations and emotions of every moment. This entire moment's reality is packed away in our memories. We know how this ends.

But for the person with Alzheimer's, there' no following moments of reality because the hall of memories spins without control every few seconds opening who knows where. The saddest part is the forgetting of the lifelong skills like swallowing, walking, and going to the bathroom. These remain longer, likely because we are hardwired to be able to do these things. Thank heavens that we cannot live very long in this brain tempest of realities and confusion. Thank God that we can paint our once loved child's name using the clouds who only days before was just another unfamiliar person in a disparate world.

I share this gift knowing that some people will call me a liar. There's no proof of the cloud writing, no sensational books where this has happened before. It happened to me, and I cherish the thought that if you look, it (or something like it) may happen for you too. Take comfort in the thought that your loved one is now doing what they love best in a perfect place from which we all come. God.

Appendices

THE FOLLOWING FIVE examples of Helen's handwriting and syntax reveal a slow, deterioration of her mental processes. Helen left hundreds of notes like these around the house before she entered a nursing home.

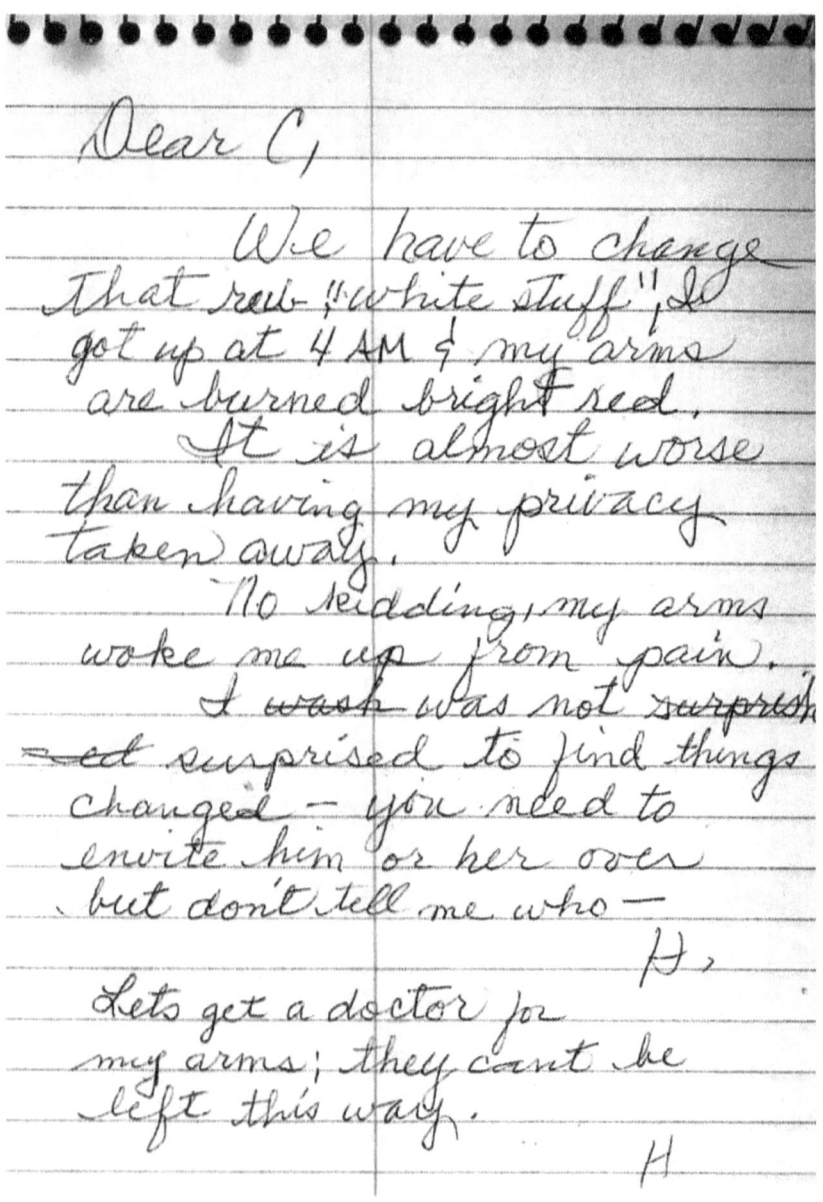

Dear C,

We have to change That red "white stuff", I got up at 4 AM & my arms are burned bright red.

It is almost worse than having my privacy taken away.

No kidding, my arms woke me up from pain.

I wash was not surprised ed surprised to find things changed — you need to invite him or her over but don't tell me who —

A,

Lets get a doctor for my arms; they cant be left this way.

H

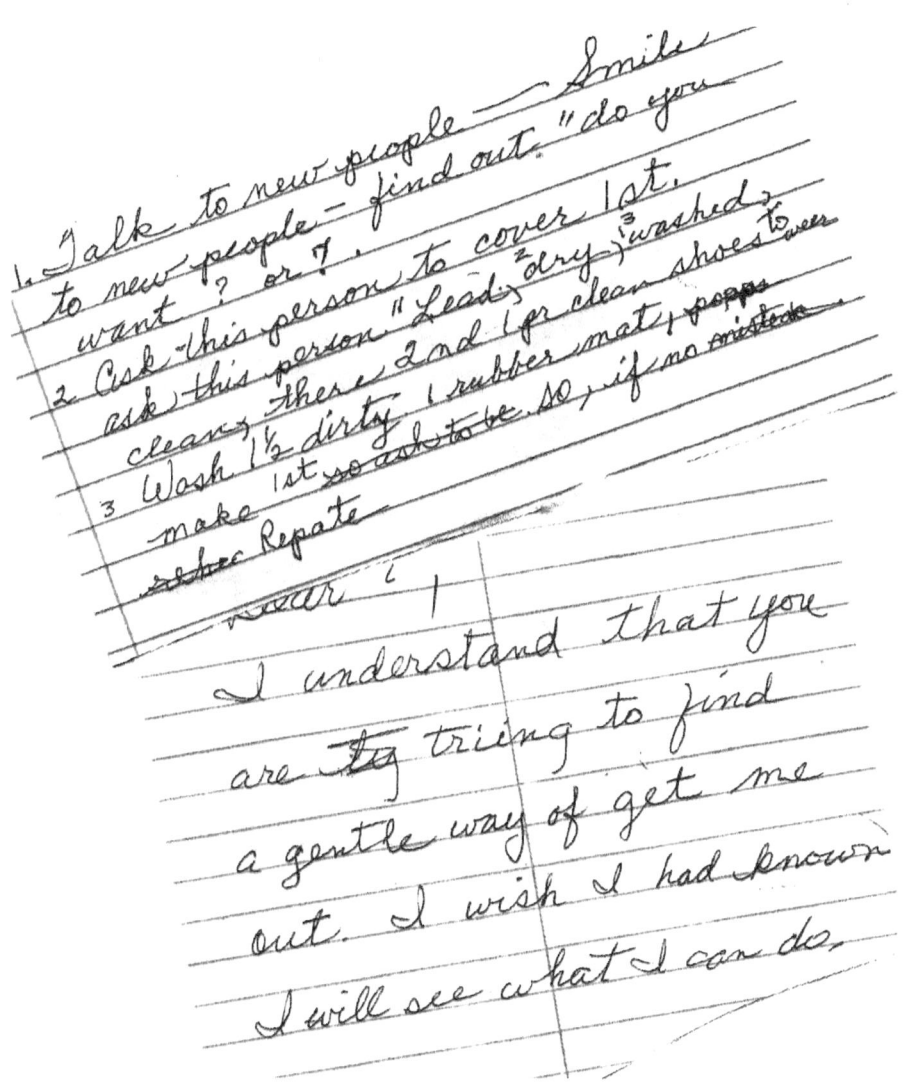

1. Talk to new people — Smile to new people - find out. "do you want ? or ?.

2. Ask "this person to cover 1st. ask this person "Lead, 2dry, 3washed, cleans, there 2nd for clean shoes over

3 Wash 1½ dirty (rubber mat, make 1st so ask to be so, if no mistake Repate

~~over~~ ?

I understand that you are ~~tr~~ trieing to find a gentle way of get me out. I wish I had known I will see what I can do.

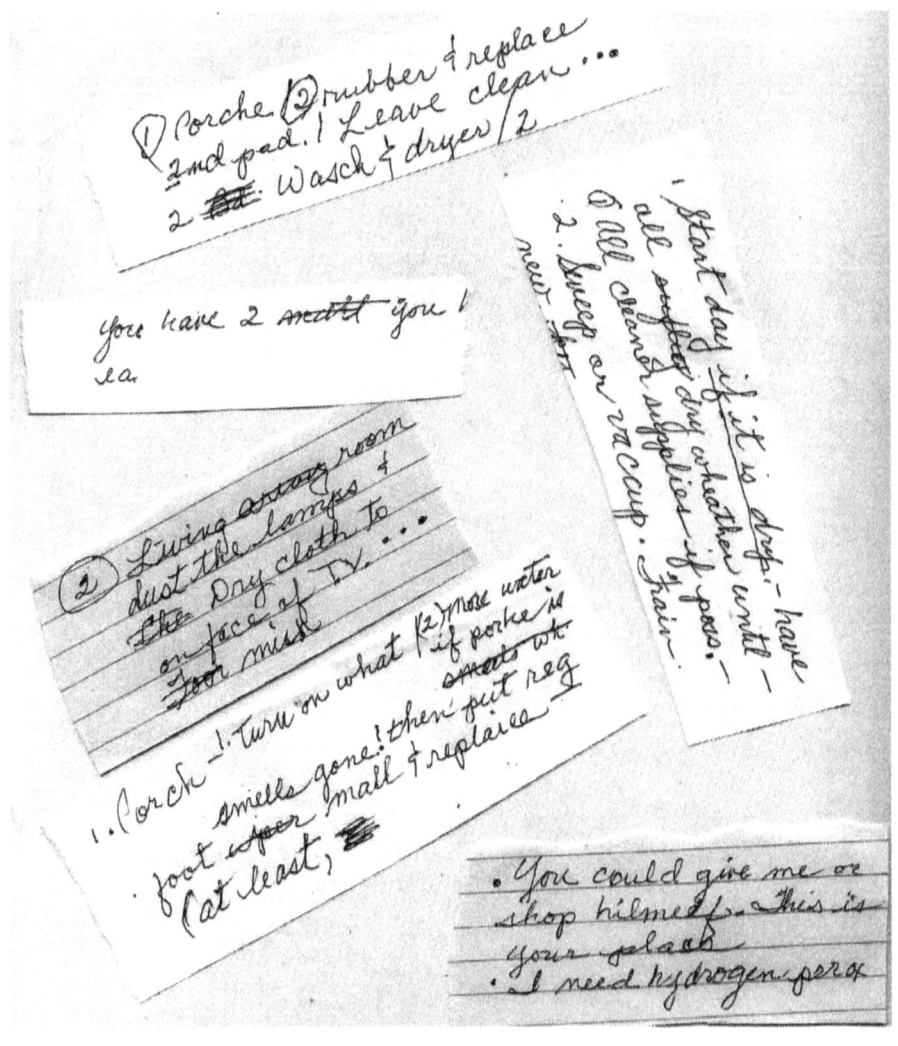

Please get me some ~~and~~
~~and~~ ~~sandwich~~ ~~ham~~ in
package — more Tomdoes

the to menti to get chell every small
samtenmooring with wibeff — all to to
menstern the smam, I by prips tring
ressh took men other others are is trying
ill tiquic monmontgoto eart most for other
jusq, so they will make ing recehing.

to to sooof/stipe to to may, more jouns-
to stoop the lurry off being too fast
jugly, Reg with ebbing this

Shotrot inos — Loon's pepley, One of th,
ople called loper whilp geanl 'it has stp
tater. I went they com bad 'Ill pell on
tonnhoo so whi com non his gica -

About The Authors

CHARLES R. McCAIN, PhD, is a retired professor of writing and English who completed his doctorate at Texas A&M University. He worked for two daily newspapers and taught photography at two universities. McCain is a sixth generation Texan. He resides in north Texas, where he has lived most of his life.

Celeste Barefield, RN, BSN, is pursuing her master's degree in nursing at Chamberlain College of Nursing, where she is specializing in hospice nursing. Newly married, Barefield has three grown children, two grandchildren, and three dachshunds. She hopes this book will guide others as they care for a family member with Alzheimer's disease and reassure them that they are not alone in their struggles and sadness.

www.ingramcontent.com/pod-product-compliance
Lightning Source LLC
Chambersburg PA
CBHW021439170526
45164CB00001B/306